On Your Terms

On Your Terms

Gender Transition Redefined for Adults

Dr. Natalia P. Zhikhareva

ISBN 979-8-9880064-6-6 (paperback)
ISBN 979-8-9880064-0-4 (ebook)
DR Z Consulting, LLC
Copyedited and Proofread by Tara Solomon
Cover design by Marko Polic
drzphd.com

Contents

ON YOUR TERMS

To my father, Peter, who never saw the gifts of his sacrifice. Dad, it was all worth it.

To find yourself, think for yourself.

— Socrates

Introduction

This book is written for adults who know that their gender identity is transgender or nonbinary.

But 100% certainty is not required here, and if you think you are trans or nonbinary but aren't fully sure, this book is also for you.

It is also for those who are thinking, contemplating, or desiring to go through gender transition but feel uncertain or afraid. And if you personally don't plan on gender transition or think it won't be worth it for you, given your circumstances, that's valid too.

It is for those who want to pass and those who don't give a shit about passing; those who prefer labels and those who do not.

Most importantly, it is for those of you who know who you are but feel scared to own it and need a tender, loving push forward.

I am here to push you. I am here to dispel stories you have been telling yourself that have kept you stuck and deeply unhappy.

Above all, I am here to empower you to craft your own terms of living authentically!

There is no one way to embody, experience, and express one's gender identity. There is only *your* way.

A note on terminology. Language is constantly evolving, especially in gender-diverse communities. Throughout the book, the terms "transgender" and "nonbinary" are used as umbrella terms to symbolize the inclusion of various gender identities.

With love and gratitude,

Dr. Z.

If you are not living your life for yourself, then who is going to live it for you?

— Ichiro Kishimi

REALITY SNIPPETS

Chapter 1

What is Gender Dysphoria?

Gender dysphoria describes psychological distress resulting from an incongruence between one's gender that was assigned at birth and one's gender identity. Many adults experienced gender dysphoria distress in childhood, while others report experiencing distress pre- or post-puberty and some later in their adult years.

The idea that gender dysphoria onset must begin at an early age of 3 or 4 is no longer held true. Clinicians today understand and witness variability in the age of onset across developmental ages.

Gender identity is not a mental health problem, however, the symptoms stemming from gender dysphoria distress are psychological in nature. Common symptoms are depression, anxiety, isolation, dissociation, body dysmorphia, and suicidal ideation.

Apart from the age of onset, many experience gender dysphoria distress ranging from mild to severe and it can fluctuate day to day, week to week, month to month, and year to year.

Some people experience gender dysphoria to such a severe extent that they are unable to function in their daily lives. Others adopt a variety of unhealthy coping mechanisms such as overworking, alcohol and drug abuse, overeating, dissociating, and isolating themselves from others and the world.

With symptoms overlapping, it becomes challenging to properly diagnose gender dysphoria, as many symptoms may cover up the root issue. For this reason, many continue to go undiagnosed and spend their time treating misdiagnosed issues in psychotherapy.

The reverse is also true, especially in young adults. What may appear as gender dysphoria is masking a deeper issue(s) that is not being addressed.

For this reason, diagnosing gender dysphoria can be as easy as a single psychological assessment and as complex as a series of ongoing therapeutic sessions.

The goal here is to listen to the patient and to exercise one's clinical discernment in asking the right questions to help the patient navigate the inner exploration of the self.

Chapter 2

What is Gender Identity?

S imply put, gender identity is your subjective sense of the self in relationship to gender. The self is defined as the totality of who you are, consisting of all characteristics and attributes; conscious and unconscious, mental, and physical.

If you were to view the self as a pizza representing your personal identity, gender identity would represent a slice of that pie. It is important to note that the self is composed of various aspects of oneself, gender being one part.

While gender identity is a single part of the whole self, it tends to carry more weight in contrast to the other parts of who you are. That's because gender identity is felt internally as your relationship to the self, subject to subject, as well as externally, how the self is perceived by others, subject to object.

Living in a world where your body, behaviors, interests, dress style, and even your patterns of speech are being gendered puts more emphasis on gender identity as a whole.

This is why, if you struggle with gender dysphoria you may also struggle in other areas of your self-identity, as many facets of who you are are being affected by the distress caused by the dysphoria.

Gender identity is personal. It is internal. Gender identity is a byproduct of reconciling your body-mind relationship and the social conditions you live in, emerging from your experiences with biological attributes unique to you. It is personal, psychological experiences rooted in your subjective reality and your social environment.

Biology, psychology, and social environment affect and form your gender identity and situate you at the center of the experience, between you and your gender identity.

This explains why, for some, gender identity is fluid and interchangeable. For others, it felt more fixed and feels stable over time.

This also explains why many older adults become aware of their gender identity much later in life without traces of childhood memories. When you exist in an environment where there is no language to describe your experiences in regard to your gender identity, parts of who you are will remain dormant. Thus any shreds of dysphoria will remain dormant until your subjective experiences come into contact with them.

For these reasons, gender identity varies from person to person. Because gender identity is rooted in one's subjective experience, there is no one way to describe it. There is only your way of defining and understanding the relationship of the self, in regard to gender identity and what it means for you as an individual.

Chapter 3

The Main Ways Gender Dysphoria Manifests

Experiencing gender dysphoria and its various manifestations is painful. The most painful part about dysphoria is its unpredictable nature—one day it centers around a particular body part, and the other day it shifts its focus to social interactions.

While varying in the age of onset, gender dysphoria further varies in regard to the initial manifestation of distress, often manifesting in three main ways:

- Physical: physical distress is felt and experienced as an internal sense of misalignment with one's secondary sex characteristics and one's experienced gender identity. I refer to physical as experiencing distress primarily concerning secondary sex characteristics or body anatomy.
- Social: gender dysphoria distress arises out of experiencing inner incongruence with one's gender assigned at birth due to the ways one internally

experiences their gender identity, and the way social environment genders the individual. Social distress is felt and experienced as an internal sense of misalignment with one's gender identity and how others gender one's body, gender expression, and gender role.

- Physical and social: it is inevitable for individuals to experience both a physical and social manifestation of gender dysphoria simultaneously. It is common for individuals who start with physical distress to develop social distress. Equally, it is common to start with social distress leading to physical distress. This is due to experiencing the self from subject to subject and subject to object, often on an ongoing basis. One cannot divorce the self from the interactions of the social world.

The manifestations of gender dysphoria further vary in intensity and can range from mild to very severe and can drastically affect one's quality of life.

Chapter 4

The Unpredictable Nature of Gender Dysphoria

Gender dysphoria is a highly unpredictable psychological phenomenon. Its unpredictable nature lies in the way it shifts throughout one's body. One time, a transgender woman in one of my groups shared:

> *"Until now, I have never felt gender dysphoria toward my genitals and wasn't interested in bottom surgery. Why do I suddenly feel an increased, unbearable dysphoria and now want to have surgery?"*

As she spoke, numerous heads in the group nodded. It became quickly apparent this was a similar experience for many. Some began to share feelings of increased dysphoria toward their hips, shoulders, voice, and other personalized features.

Gender dysphoria is a nasty beast. It does not discriminate. It operates under zero logic. It moves in no detectable patterns, and it strikes its victims when they least expect it.

That's why I like to call it a silent assassin.

One of the main reasons why dysphoria shifts throughout the body is due to the dormancy effect. For example, if you are in the early stages of questioning your gender identity, a big part of your authentic self is still dormant. When you are not in touch with your authentic self, it remains asleep. Therefore, the dysphoria in relation to that part of yourself remains dormant as well.

That's why gender dysphoria tends to spike once you come out as transgender or nonbinary. The part that remained dormant is no longer asleep! Resulting in increased incongruence between how you feel on the inside and how the world perceives you.

The second main reason why gender dysphoria shifts throughout the body is due to the overall congruency you start to achieve. I know this may sound confusing. Shouldn't gender dysphoria decrease vs. increase in this case?

Well, not for everyone. Remember, gender dysphoria has zero logic and no discernible pattern to it!

What happens for many, is this: A person begins to address their gender dysphoria and decides to go through a gender transition. As they start hormones, they often feel better. Finally having the right hormone in their body. In their body, they also feel better because they are finally doing something about their gender dysphoria.

After a few months on hormones, gender dysphoria shifts to other body parts and begins to increase. For many, it could be anything; ranging from facial hair to discomfort with chest size. Often it is the physical feature that is visible to others and may lead to misgendering.

As you can see, it is an ongoing, moving target. Oscillating on one body part until congruency is achieved as it shifts again.

While this doesn't happen for everyone, those who do experience it find themselves constantly fighting the assassin that springs up on them.

Chapter 5

Effects of Gender Dysphoria on Your Life

Gender dysphoria affects everyone differently. Some people experience mild symptoms, while many others experience severe symptoms to the point of being unable to take care of themselves.

The longer you have been living with gender dysphoria, the longer you may have convinced yourself that you can continue to cope with it. Telling yourself you have managed up till now.

It's a dangerous game you continue to play with yourself because you don't realize just how harmful living with gender dysphoria really is.

The danger lies in just how much gender dysphoria occupies your mental function and the effects it has on your surroundings. When you are struggling with symptoms of dysphoria, your brain struggles to combat the dissonance between your gender assigned at birth and your desired gender.

As a result of the ongoing inner struggles, your mind devotes a tremendous amount of energy to solving what it perceives as a problem. Creating a buzzing white noise in the back of your head that never goes away. Operating in the background without your full awareness.

This buzzing noise occupies the majority of your mental function and is responsible for:

- decreased productivity at home and work
- inability to focus and concentrate on tasks in front of you
- depressed mood and affect
- inability to be present and connect to your loved ones
- difficulty falling asleep
- loss of sexual desire
- fluctuations in appetite
- detachment from your body
- ailments in your health

Do any of these sound familiar to you? These are just some of the most common symptoms stemming from the mental struggle your brain engages in.

One of the biggest dangers of gender dysphoria occupying so much of your mind is an internal shift you experience from living to existing.

What's the difference? When you are living your life, you are able to be present; savor the moment and emotionally feel and enjoy your experiences. You are more present and emotionally attuned in your daily life and around your loved ones.

When you exist, you turn into a robot. A zombie. Operating in survival mode as you try to make it, one day at a time. You become emotionally unavailable and disengaged from your loved ones. To your family and friends, you come across as withdrawn and distant.

Of course, there are glimpses of life; meeting the love of your life, the birth of your child, and personal accomplishment, but the majority of your time is spent on autopilot.

The amount of space and energy dysphoria takes to occupy your mind is not healthy! Your mind was not designed to devote 24/7 of your energy to focus on a singular problem of this magnitude.

The continuous back and forth experienced as a result of the dissonance and incongruence you feel with your gender puts tremendous strain on your psyche.

And it can, and for some people it does, break their minds.

That's why it is so important to talk to someone about gender dysphoria. Talking to someone eases up the pressure your mind is experiencing, even if you are not ready to take any steps other than acknowledging that you are struggling.

I think you can talk yourself into your dreams, or you can talk yourself out of your dreams.

I think not running your own race is probably another one of the biggest things that keeps people from their destiny. Because you can't run somebody else's race.

— Joel Osteen

STOP TELLING
YOURSELF THIS

Chapter 1

"I Can Continue to Cope with Gender Dysphoria."

Many of you confuse coping with suffering, thinking that what you do is a healthy coping skill. The truth is that gender dysphoria is not susceptible to management.

I know. Getting dark here.

While you can put a temporary bandage on it, you are still bleeding—bleeding heavily as your dysphoria drips into other areas of your life, leaving a blood splatter everywhere you go and affecting everything and everybody around you.

I know exactly what happens. You start experiencing gender dysphoria symptoms and begin ruminating whether or not you are transgender. The more you ruminate, the more you tell yourself this can't be true.

You begin to engage with suffering, masquerading as coping. Overworking yourself to death. Drinking. Overeating. Avoiding quality time with family and friends. Binge feminizing or masculinizing with clothing, only to purge later. Escaping into TV. The list is endless.

The tricky part is that your brain actually believes you are coping with gender dysphoria. It tells you:

> *"See, if this were real dysphoria, you wouldn't be able to carry on with your life as your assigned gender at birth."*

But it's a trick!

Your brain will employ a series of tricks because it knows that deep down inside, you are terrified of change. You are terrified of the potential risks moving forward can bring. But what about the benefits it can offer?

Suffering is overrated. It is unnecessary.

Coping in any shape or form disguised as suffering doesn't prove shit. It doesn't prove you are not trans, and it sure doesn't prove you can live with dysphoria. All it shows is how masochistic you are toward yourself, and that's heartbreaking because you deserve so much more than the pain you are imposing on yourself.

Stop telling yourself you can cope, and start talking to someone about the struggles you are experiencing so that you can begin healing.

Chapter 2

"I Can Solve This Problem."

Our brains are designed to solve problems. When it can't, we become anxious and stressed. And while our brains are great at solving even the most complex problems, many are not subject to solutions by mind alone.

Gender dysphoria is one of them. To begin with, it is simply not a mental problem. For this reason, this and other similar mental tactics don't work.

> *"If I just learn to cope with dysphoria better, it will disappear."*
> *"If I get married, dysphoria will go away."*
> *"If I become a parent, that proves I am not dysphoric."*
> *"I just need to join the army and embrace my assigned gender, and it will go away."*

Attempting to solve gender dysphoria simply within your headspace leads to running circles inside your head. As your mind starts working overtime, your anxiety rises. As your anxiety rises, you start getting into a catastrophizing mindset.

This is where every possible outcome appears bad, and you feel paralyzed to move forward. Finally, your mind fills up with decision fatigue and you find yourself giving up on yourself.

This is why physical and social transitions are so helpful to adults struggling with gender dysphoria. Once they start feeling more comfortable physically, the mental anguish lessens.

So stop selling yourself a lie that you can solve this problem with your mind alone. Start acknowledging that the only way to deal with this problem is to do something about it. Even if that doing is as small as sharing who you truly are with others.

Chapter 3

"I Can Outrun Gender Dysphoria."

Every day you wake up, you put your running-coping shoes on, hoping to outrun gender dysphoria.

There is no doubt about it; it is a race. A nasty one. A race you keep losing every single time. A race with one marked winner, and it's not you.

It is a race of denial. A race you continue to engage in, thinking what's happening within you is not happening to you.

Denial is a losing game. It doesn't last. You can't win at denial. Sure, it may feel safe to remain in denial. To avoid confronting that which you fear. But eventually, that which you refuse to acknowledge comes up to the surface and when it does, it's never pretty.

Remember, what you resist, persists!

If this were a race you could win, millions would opt out of gender transition. Because let's face it, gender transition is not easy and carries financial, emotional, and social challenges.

Stop trying to outrun gender dysphoria. It is faster, mightier, and has a better pair of shoes to run in. It has years of experience under its belt of outrunning humans. It is unbeatable.

The only way to beat it is to stop running. To stop living in denial. To acknowledge and accept it. Take control of your life and take steps to minimize or eliminate gender dysphoria altogether.

Stop wasting your precious time. Time is an asset you can't get more of. Nor can you get your time back.

So stop. Learn how to confront it, accept it, and decide if there are steps you can take to better your quality of life. And it doesn't have to be giant scary steps such as starting gender transition. Gender transition is not mandatory and is not for everyone.

You can start by refusing to run the race. Take the running shoes off, acknowledge that you are struggling with gender dysphoria, and end the denial.

Chapter 4

"I Can't Handle Gender Transition."

I f gender transition is something you desire, I bet the thought of not being able to handle transition crossed your mind more than once. At the core of that thought is fear, and part of the fear is the stories you tell yourself.

"Everyone will leave me if I transition."
"If I transition, I will be ugly."
"My spouse will divorce me."
"I will lose my job."
"My life will be destroyed."
"I will lose everything I worked so hard for."
"Society won't ever see me as my true gender."
"What if I make a mistake?"
"What if I am really losing my mind or making this up?"
"What if I realize I am not trans?"

Sometimes the stories you tell yourself are films projected on the big screen. Each one plays on repeat, again and again, and as each movie repeats, your fears increase.

I am not saying that some of these fear-based thoughts don't actually come true for some people. They do. That's the reality of going through a dramatic life event.

What I want you to realize is that your fears are not literally about any of these things. It may feel as if it is, but it isn't.

The surface level of the fear that you perceive as real is covering up a subconscious root cause. When you say you fear others won't support you, that's a surface fear. Underneath it is a deeper reason why you feel afraid.

Your fears are always tied to the subconscious root cause. Let me share with you what lies subconsciously underneath all these fears.

If you take a shovel and dig deep into your subconscious, you'll find a single constant denominator beneath all your fears: you are afraid you won't be able to handle it. It's a fear of being unable to handle whatever comes your way.

- Fear of being abandoned. You are afraid you won't be able to handle it.
- Fear of losing your job. You are afraid you won't be able to handle it.
- Fear of not passing. You are afraid you won't be able to handle it.

Do you see the common denominator that unites all of these fears? There is only one and it's all about feeling afraid you won't be able to handle things.

Here is what you need to know about the fear of not being able to handle it: you are an adult! That means you have lived some portion of your life. Maybe you are in your 20s, 30s, 40s, 50s, or even 80s.

You lived that much. That means you have been capable of taking care of yourself. Sustaining a job. Paying your bills. Taking care of your household. Some of you have been responsible for your kids, spouses, and parents.

Notice how you have been handling a lot of things throughout your life! I bet a lot of them were scary at first. I bet you felt like you couldn't handle them. I bet there were many times you felt you would fail.

But you didn't. You took steps forward despite feeling fearful, and you realized you could handle it! And once you were able to handle it, the fear went away. Isn't that interesting? You see, once you get a handle on it, you no longer feel scared.

Many of you seldom realize that you have been handling so much of your life on top of living with gender dysphoria.

Handling gender dysphoria in the best capacity you could, without completely falling apart, is incredibly difficult.

If you have been handling all of those years while struggling with gender dysphoria, what makes you think you can't handle this?

Trust me, you are more resilient than you realize and have all the inner resources you need to handle stepping into your gender identity!

Chapter 5

"If I Transition, I Will Look Ugly."

Many have shared with me their fear of becoming unattractive if they go through a gender transition. This fear is often heard from trans women or feminine nonbinary folks but is also seen in trans men and masculine nonbinary people.

One of the reasons why this fear is seen in feminine individuals is because society places a high bar on what women should look like. There is also a lot of pressure and emphasis to pass and to look a particular way within the transgender community itself. If you do not meet "community standards," you quickly become branded as someone who is not working on their transition.

Additionally, society is quick to dehumanize, shame, and tear down transfeminine people if they do not live up to their view of what a woman should look like. Quick to humiliate. To point out that trans women can never be women. That they will always look like a man pretending to be a woman.

Trans men and masculine nonbinary folks get similar treatment, although I see this less frequently. Being judged that they do not live up to the ideal of a man, whatever that may be. Having their masculinity scrutinized and put on public display. Emasculated by the idea that one can never have a "real penis" and, therefore, can never be a man.

To all that, I say, "fuck society and fuck community standards!"

To you, I pose this question:

> *"Would you rather be attractive, but miserable, in your gender assigned at birth?"*

or

> *"Would you rather be unattractive, but healthy and happy, in your authentic gender?"*

I also want you to ponder the idea of what is perceived as attractive and unattractive. As well, realize that the person you are now, the one who is feeling afraid of not measuring up to the ideal of beauty, is not the same person you will become.

Once you start taking steps toward your authentic self, you'll feel happier. Your overall health and well-being will improve and with that improvement, a new perspective arises as you realize how much happier you are.

When you experience this perspective shift, your perception of what you fear will change. Including the high bar you have set for yourself.

Chapter 6

"I Must be Losing My Mind."

When people start working with me, one of the questions many ask is:

"Am I losing my mind?"

The truth is, when you are living with gender dysphoria, it is common to feel like you are losing your mind. To start believing that your mind is making dysphoria up. To begin searching for other reasons to help you rationalize how you feel.

One of the reasons why you feel like you are losing your mind is because your mind is struggling to close the dissonance gap between your life experiences and your gender identity.

Many of you have been overcompensating with your gender assignment by engaging in gender-stereotypical activities:

- joining the military
- becoming the captain of your football team

- joining a sorority
- becoming a beauty queen

When you have lived your life pretending who you are to such an extent, your brain starts to believe this must be who you are. As you begin to get in touch with your authentic gender, the distance in the dissonance gap is hard to ignore.

The dissonance gap breeds anxiety, leading to you thinking you are losing your mind. And while you may not think you are losing your mind in a mental health crisis way, many of you describe what you experience as a feeling of your mind losing its grip on reality.

If you still believe you are losing your mind, let me ask you, are you able to care for yourself daily?

Shower? Dress? Eat? Go to work and hold a job? Shop for groceries or order in? Come home and take your dog out? Get on your cell phone and browse social media — post comments and reply back?

If you answered yes to any of the above, you are far saner than you realize. Now I get it; dysphoria will do this. It will create a mirage, a constant fog around you to obscure your clarity of vision and your clarity of thinking.

At some point, you will be scratching your head, if not already, wondering if you are absolutely losing your mind. Insane to even consider trans identity, thinking that you must be detached from reality to even contemplate gender transition.

Don't let dysphoria mess with your sanity by creating the deception of insanity. Remember, it's all a mirage.

· · ·

mi·rage

noun

noun: **mirage**; plural noun: **mirages**

1. an optical illusion caused by atmospheric conditions, especially the appearance of a sheet of water in something that appears real or possible but is not in fact so.

2. something that appears real or possible but is not in fact so.

Stop telling yourself you are losing your mind! You are not.

Chapter 7

"I'll End Up Like Others Who Have Destransitioned."

OK! The elephant is in the room! Yes, people do detransition. Detransition involves discontinuing or reversing some or all aspects of gender transition. Detransition happens, and we are still in the very early research of trying to lay out patterns as to why.

People detransition for various personal reasons, some of which are:

- past mental health histories led to feelings of gender dysphoria
- health concerns associated with hormone treatment
- negative effects of medical and surgical treatment
- gender identity evolved beyond what they thought it was
- gender transition did not resolve gender dysphoria
- gender transition is too stigmatizing and too difficult
- lack of support from others

These reasons and many others are all valid concerns to take gender transition seriously. And if you are considering going through some elements of gender transition, I highly recommend considering all the pros and cons.

Gender transition is life-changing, and it is important to ensure it is the right decision for you. While many prefer going through medical and surgical transitions, it's important to emphasize it's not mandatory.

One common thread among the individuals who decided to detransition is that each story is deeply individual and personal.

So is your story! Your story of gender evolution is rooted in your individuality and is situated in your personal history, circumstances, and most importantly, your gender goals.

Comparing your potential to a personal decision someone else had to make about detransition is robbing yourself of an opportunity to thrive. While it is important to listen to the stories of people who have gone through a detransition, it is equally important not to equate their fate with yours!

Remember, people decide to detransition for numerous reasons. Assuming the same will happen to you is assuming your history, circumstances, and personal relationship to your gender are identical.

Chapter 8

"I Need More Information."

I t is natural to lean toward information when you start questioning your gender identity or wondering if you struggle with gender dysphoria.

To become obsessive by your search for *the* right answer you seek. To watch numerous YouTube videos. Listen to a gazillion podcasts. And follow every transgender's personal social media account.

Sure, information is important! Having some idea of what gender transition entails is a must. Consulting with a mental health provider to confirm gender dysphoria is essential. Sitting down with a doctor to gather more intel before deciding on hormones is vital. Having a consultation with a gender-affirming surgeon and going over all the pros and cons is indispensable.

What you don't need is to become an information *hoarder*!

You tell yourself you'll begin when all the information is collected, stalling your transition and life by lying to yourself, convincing your mind you are being smart and prudent by making sure you know all there is to know about dysphoria and gender transition. As the years pass, and you still haven't taken a single step forward, you still find yourself struggling with gender dysphoria.

"But information is power!"

No. It is not. Information is *potential power*. Power is what you do. Not how much you know. Stop telling yourself you need more information. Chances are, you already have all the info you need.

Start taking small steps, even as small as acknowledging to yourself that you have gender dysphoria and need to make an appointment with a professional to confirm it. But please, start today.

Chapter 9

"My Partner Won't Let Me Transition."

I f you are in a relationship or a marriage and feel you can't start a gender transition because your partner will leave you, you are engaging in self-sabotage.

If your partner gave you an ultimatum:

> *"If you transition, I leave, and the marriage (relationship) is over."*

And if you are clinging to it, you are also engaging in self-sabotage.

I know that it may not feel like a self-sabotage tactic to you. And while it may not "feel" like it, it is. Self-sabotage is an unconscious defense you engage in to avoid feeling abandoned.

Many of you, if not most, who are struggling with gender dysphoria have a deep unconscious fear of being unlovable; that people will leave you and you will end up all alone.

Feelings of abandonment are a byproduct of years of living with gender dysphoria and, as a result, internalizing feelings of guilt and shame. These feelings of guilt and shame lead you to create an inner dialogue that if anyone knew your identity, they would never love you for who you truly are.

Chances are, you tend to overcompensate with people you have been in a relationship with, often by taking on too many responsibilities. This might appear as subconsciously catering to their needs while denying yours, or overvaluing others around you and devaluing yourself.

It is natural as a self-preservation defense to unconsciously choose to stay with the person when they offer an ultimatum. After all, this is what you taught yourself to believe. It is also common to continue to neglect your physical and mental health by not addressing gender dysphoria and acquiescing to your partner's ultimatum.

And as painful as it is to hear, your partner does not hold you hostage! You do!

You are your own terrorist, holding yourself in this position, terrorizing your own decisions because you have gotten accustomed to overcompensating out of fear of abandonment.

Trust me, it pains me to be so upfront with you, but you deserve to hear the truth. The way to freedom is through understanding the patterns of behaviors that hold you hostage. Self-sabotage is one of them, and it can be challenging to break this pattern, but it is possible.

If you are telling yourself you can't, won't, and mustn't transition because of your partner, please at the very least realize it is you, not them, who is holding yourself tied up in bondage by continuing to engage in self-sabotage.

Chapter 10

"Fear is a Sign I Will Fail."

Fear is a big one when it comes to gender transition. While there are a lot of valid reasons for it, there are equally, if not more, exaggerated ones.

Let's unpack fear. Fear has two faces. The first face is fear of real physical danger. You know you must trust and listen to this fear when you experience a physical reaction. This reaction is known as a flight or fight response.

A classic example is walking down a street and encountering a lion. OK, an unlikely occurrence, but humor me here. When you see a lion, your body goes into a flight response as your brain signals you to run for your life. We all need to trust and listen to that kind of fear because it is there to protect us.

The second type of fear is fear of the unknown. This type of fear occurs in about 90% of your situations and always has to do with fearing whom you want to be and what you want to do. More precisely, it is fear that you won't be able to handle new things, changes, and environments.

This is the primary fear orbiting your desire to explore your gender identity or to start taking steps toward gender transition.

I know you know these fears all too well because you wake up and go to sleep with them every single day. It follows you around like an abandoned puppy begging to be adopted.

It begs to be part of your life because this is a good kind of fear. Yes, I know I said "good"! The kind of fear that you should embrace because it wants to make positive, lasting changes in your life.

One of the ways you can tell it's a good kind of fear is if you continue to find yourself thinking, fantasizing, or daydreaming about yourself in your authentic gender vs. gender assigned at birth but feel afraid to do anything about it.

Think back on other times when you wanted to do something but felt afraid. For me, it was writing this book, and believe me, the fear was there. Every day I woke up thinking about how I wanted to get this book out there and feeling terrified at the same time. It wasn't until I acknowledged that fear was not the problem that I learned how to move forward with my dreams in spite of it. I am forever grateful I was able to befriend my fear and that you are now holding my book in your hands.

Imagine what changes can happen in your life if you befriend your fears. If you moved forward, closer to your true gender in spite of feeling afraid.

I am not going to tell you to stop being afraid because that's not always possible. But what is possible is to trust that the fear is there to help nudge you forward.

One of the ways you can begin working on trusting this fear is to recognize how much it has to do with what you desire. If you continue to think about something you want, don't you think it's worth investigating what that want tells you?

Learning to trust this fear is different from behaving impulsively, rashly, or without thinking. On the contrary, it is about slowing down and paying attention to the changes you want to make in your life but feel afraid to.

To work on your trust, I recommend writing down all the pros and cons you can think of about what you fear. Writing things down helps you to look at your fears more objectively as you remove them from the busy chatter of your mind. This allows you to realistically consider the pros and cons without the catastrophizing, fear-based thoughts that tend to ruminate inside of your head.

Begin working on learning how to walk forward despite fear, and when you do that, your life begins to change drastically!

A lot of people will tell you what you want to achieve can't be done.

Never internalize their limits as your own.

— Russ

CONSIDER THIS

Chapter 1

Learn to Separate Internal vs. External Fears

Fears are an inevitable part of your evolution toward your authentic self. The more you know and understand your fears, the better equipped you will be to make life-changing decisions related to your gender identity.

Remember, fear is not an obstacle you need to overcome but more of a signpost you need to pay attention to. Oftentimes, fear is a good sign. Other times, it's there to offer you more information to aid you in the right direction.

Spotting the difference between internal vs. external fear becomes especially instrumental when you explore your gender identity or make the decision to gender transition.

In these instances, fears will almost always be there. This is a normal and natural reaction to have, especially since you are about to undergo a major change in your life. Many of your fears may fall into various categories:

- afraid of making a mistake

- afraid of losing loved ones
- afraid of not passing
- afraid of not being able to find a partner
- afraid you won't be accepted
- afraid you'll have a medical complication

While these fears may appear different on the surface, I have observed that they fall into two main categories.

The first category of fear revolves around the internal aspect of the self. Often this internalized fear is expressed as:

"I am afraid I will make a mistake."

or

"I am afraid I will realize I am not transgender."

This fear is related to the inner uncertainty you are experiencing regarding your relationship to your gender identity. You may feel unsure about your gender identity and not fully confident that you are transgender or nonbinary.

And that's OK! Gender identity is incredibly complex, and it can take time to fully understand what your personal relationship to your gender is. Uncertainty is more common for people who have not experienced gender dysphoria dating back to childhood. The lack of earlier experiences adds confusion to the mix as you begin to wonder if you truly are trans.

What I want you to know is that fear related to uncertainty about who you are is simply telling you that you are unsure. It can be an indicator that you may need to:

- spend more time exploring your gender identity
- engage in a safe exploration of your gender, such as social transition, before taking steps toward medical or surgical transition
- or seek the support of a gender therapist to further process the underlying causes of the fear

Over decades of experience working with transgender adults, I have often seen internalized fears of uncertainty toward self-identity or fear of making a mistake more in younger adults ages 18–25; this is less likely in older adults, but it still happens.

In my experience, individuals who are sure of their transgender identity and know they want to undergo gender transition seldom experience this category of fear, although it is possible.

If you find yourself experiencing internalized fears of this nature, it may be a good indicator to pause and explore your relationship with your gender. This will enable you to feel more affirmed and confident about your gender identity and be more assertive to take steps toward gender transition.

The second category of fear related to starting a gender transition revolves around exterior situations, representing externalized fears. Often these fears are expressed as:

"I am afraid I won't pass if I transition."

or

"I am afraid I will lose my loved one."

This fear reflects your sense of self and ability to handle external events. In contrast to internalized fears, this type of fear does not call into question your inner sense of gender identity.

Instead, these fears are rooted in your ability, or feeling lack thereof, to handle what may happen if you decide to undergo a gender transition. As a result, the externalized type of fear keeps you stuck as you fear going forward and potentially confronting that which you fear.

If you experience this fear, it may be a good indicator to ensure you have all your ducks in order before starting the gender transition. Make sure your support system is set up. Ensure you have people around you who can be there for you.

If there isn't anyone in your personal life to elicit support, is there a local community you can rely on? If not, what about online groups and online support?

What are the other ducks you need to consider? Make a list of all the things you are concerned about and try as best as possible to set up a plan to address them. Addressing your external fears by thinking about solutions to potential problems you fear will help you feel more confident to move forward. It will also make you feel more in control of the potential future.

Chapter 2

Trust Your Inner Compass

As adults, many of you have been living and struggling with gender dysphoria for several years. Some of you even managed to cope for a decade or two! In my opinion, you are all experts on gender dysphoria in your own right.

Why is it that, when it comes to your own sense of gender identity, you are so quick to disregard and dismiss years of experiences? And quick to assume your mind is making it up or that dysphoria will suddenly disappear one day?

Some of you are quick to trust the internet, social influencers, or the world when it comes to your gender identity over your own long-term experiences. And while youngsters may need guidance about their gender identity, you, as an adult with lived experiences, have a better inner compass about who you are!

I know it can be challenging to trust yourself, especially if you have spent a lot of time in denial. Or when your family or your partner tells you otherwise. When the world is quick to dismiss your reality as truth! To top it off, you may also experience internal and external fears, making it much harder to trust yourself.

If you lost touch with your inner compass, taking affirming steps toward your inner truth helps.

What exactly are affirming steps? Affirming steps are little steps set up on your way to your gender exploration. Each step builds on the prior one as you become more confident in your gender identity.

One of the biggest benefits of taking affirming steps is the certainty each step offers in ensuring you are moving in the right direction. If your steps affirm how you identify, you know you are on the right track and can move forward. If not, it could indicate that you need more time to explore your gender.

Affirming steps are also a great way to help you increase strength and resilience against naysayers around you. With each step, your confidence will grow, leading to a stronger, more resilient self.

Some of the affirming steps to consider:

- journaling how you feel about your gender identity
- sharing your feelings with a person you trust
- expressing yourself in your authentic gender by changing your appearance
- changing your name and pronouns
- creating a vision board of how you see yourself in your true gender
- coming out

- attending a local support group
- working with a gender therapist
- making an appointment with a gender-affirming doctor to obtain information on the pros and cons of hormone therapy

Chapter 3

Get Your Own Cookie Cutter

Out of all the identities underneath the transgender and nonbinary umbrella, it can be confusing to figure out which gender identity fits you.

Are you:

- Trans man
- Trans woman
- Trans masculine
- Trans feminine
- Genderqueer
- Androgyne
- Genderfluid

And these are just a few of the many gender identities present today.

When trying to figure out your gender identity, it can be easy to get lost in the voices of others; your family, partner, and friends, as they chime in on what your gender identity is.

Today especially, everyone, including the media, has an opinion on what your gender is and whether you should or should not consider gender transition. Suddenly it feels like everyone is an expert on your personal and internal sense of self and are eager to tell you what your gender is and how you should identify, present, and express yourself.

I hope you realize how unrealistic and ridiculous the concept of someone knowing you better than you know yourself is. Not only is it unrealistic, but it is also impossible.

That's why it is important to find your cookie cutter; the cookie cutter that better resonates with you and carve out your own cookie, a.k.a. how you identify.

Your cookie's shape, texture, and flavor are based on your goals, needs, wants, and life circumstances. Your cookie may also be mutable. Changing as you change and grow. Shifting and taking on a different shape as you step further and further into your own self. It may also be fixed and remain the same amazing chocolate chip forever.

The more you explore your gender identity, the better you are at knowing what your cookie flavor and shape are.

When you listen to too many voices about your identity, you invite too many bakers into your kitchen! Each one is eager to use their cookie cutter to define who you are. To carve out the shape they think you should be.

Stop letting other bakers into your kitchen! Start trusting your inner knowing as you take steps to explore and affirm what you know.

Chapter 4

Build Houses Not Castles

I hear a lot of anxiety-driven feelings when people start out on their path.

"I will come out when I feel confident."
"I will tell my family I am on hormones when I start feeling better."
"I will go out there into the world as myself only when I feel I pass."

These feelings indicate inner resistance to change because many of you don't want to change. Let's be honest, there is much about change that we all want to avoid.

For starters, change feels uncomfortable as it pushes you outside of your comfort zone. Additionally, change brings along responsibilities you want to avoid confronting.

That's where resistance comes in and a big part of coping with resistance is telling yourself that you'll take steps forward once you feel more confident and secure.

In this case, once you do feel more confident and secure, you are more likely to move forward through the resistance.

The question is: How to cultivate this confidence? This is where my analogy of building houses, and not castles, comes in.

Imagine you are sitting on the floor surrounded by Legos. Each Lego represents a step toward your gender exploration or gender transition.

- A Lego for becoming aware of who you are
- A Lego for your first session with the therapist or a visit to a gender-affirming clinic
- A Lego for finding your name
- A Lego for starting to express how you see yourself
- A Lego for starting hormones

Sitting on the floor, you begin to stack up your wins by building up your first Lego castle. Every step, no matter how small, is a win you achieved. With every win, your confidence grows as you prove to yourself you can handle it; that you have inner strengths and resilience to own who you are despite of any obstacles and fears.

As your confidence builds, your castle grows taller. Suddenly you begin to feel afraid to share your castle with others, fearing they will tear it down with their words, looks, or glances.

The desire to hide what you have built intensifies. To protect yourself, you continue building your castle in private, waiting for self-assurance to pump you up so that you feel braver to come out.

Until one day, you stand back and admire your castle. Feeling confident and proud of your accomplishments, you feel ready to share your castle with the world.

Sadly, for many people, their castle gets shattered. It gets knocked to the ground by other people's reactions and their inner projections of whom they want you to be.

As your castle plummets, so does your confidence. This is often a time when many decide to call it quits. They stop taking steps toward themselves. They stop exploring their gender identity. And they stop going through gender transition.

The shattering of everything you have built privately is too much to bear. Feelings of guilt and shame that surface may spiral you into repressing your identity, locking your authentic self deep inside of you.

Perhaps you have already experienced your castle being crushed by the weight of others' projections, prejudice, and hatred. Perhaps you are familiar with the pain and hurt that follows along with a desire to hide from the world.

But what if I told you, it is possible to maintain your confidence even if others crush your Lego castle?

The secret to this is learning how to build tiny houses, not a castle! And if you feel too defeated to start again, I promise you, there is more strength within you than you realize.

When you build a castle, you are putting all of the energy of your hopes and dreams into one foundation. Stacking your wins privately until your castle is tall enough to give you the confidence you need to share yourself with others. By doing this, you are placing all of your expectations and all of your bets onto your single castle. This is just like putting all of your eggs into one basket.

When your castle gets smashed, you feel defeated and discouraged to start again. Hopeless to pursue your dreams. Insecure to move forward.

Here is my secret: Start building small houses of individual wins, and soon enough, you will have an entire city. Start sharing each house with everyone around you instead of keeping it a secret. Stop waiting to feel confident until you are ready to share. Realize confidence comes with sharing, showing up, and owning who you are!

If any of your houses get smashed, take a deep breath. Look around and realize your city is still standing strong. You are surrounded by other wins you have made.

As you begin rebuilding any broken houses, your confidence will soar as you show yourself how resourceful you are. You will begin to witness your ability to get up and confront any damage your city has sustained.

With every rebuild, your foundation becomes stronger and more resilient. You can sustain future attacks on your houses because you have already emotionally experienced them. Been there, done that!

That is confidence! Confidence arises out of your perseverance, and the only way to get there is to learn how to build small houses instead of giant castles.

Chapter 5

Criticism is Always Up for Sale

Unsolicited advice, anyone? Welcome to the world of gender, where everybody has something to say about your gender identity in the form of unsolicited advice masqueraded as positive feedback.

Interestingly, their feedback is seldom in the form of affirmation, support, or encouragement. It is often in the form of criticism.

> *"Are you sure you know your gender because I don't*
> *recall seeing any of this from you before?" a.k.a.*
> *"You don't know shit about yourself."*
> *"You are being brainwashed by social media." a.k.a.*
> *"You are a naive idiot who can't think for*
> *yourself."*
> *"I don't think it's going to work out for you." a.k.a.*
> *"You being you is going to ruin your life."*

The list of criticism is endless. What you need to know about criticism masquerading as unsolicited advice is that it's cheap! It's free! And it has zero value because it's crap!

Certainly, constructive criticism exists and can be instrumental in exploring who you are. The key is distinguishing where the feedback is coming from and whether a person offering it is qualified to give it.

Brené Brown said:

 If you aren't in the arena getting your ass kicked on occasion, I am not interested in or open to your feedback. There are a million cheap seats in the world today filled with people who will never be brave with their own lives, but will spend every ounce of energy they have hurling dice and judgment at those of us trying to dare greatly. Their only contributions are criticism, cynicism, and fear-mongering. If you're criticizing from a place where you're not also putting yourself on the line, I'm not interested in your feedback.

The next time you hear someone criticizing you, ask yourself if they are in the arena with you. Are they people who genuinely mean you well? Are they providers who have experience working with transgender and nonbinary folks?

If the answer is no, realize that not every feedback is valid.

Chapter 6

The Illusion of Social Acceptance

When you struggle with self-acceptance of who you are and have difficulty validating your identity, you begin seeking that validation from others through social acceptance.

Many feel a need to be accepted by cis people, hoping that will validate their gender identity. Others are compelled to be socially accepted by their society or culture to feel validated. And some seek validation from strangers on social platforms.

When you seek validation from others before you can validate yourself, you appear socially insecure and unsure. This insecurity signals uncertainty to others around you. When others are uncertain about your gender identity, they will assume what it is, and their assumptions are often entangled with their projections. In doing this, you are relying on the projections of how others see your gender identity.

Whenever you struggle to validate yourself, you wait for your family, friends, or partner to validate you. In doing this, you are waiting for them to choose you. Every time you wait for someone to befriend you on social media or to like your post, you are also waiting for them to choose you.

When you seek validation from others, you are creating a co-dependency based on that need. When social acceptance is not given, you start feeling unloved, unwanted, and unseen.

The self-loathing you may already feel toward yourself after years of living with dysphoria and telling yourself you are unworthy intensifies with the negative self-perception of being rejected by others. This becomes a vicious self-fulfilling prophecy of your life.

You do all of this to feel socially accepted. What you don't realize is that by letting others choose you before you can choose yourself, puts you at the mercy of their personal beliefs and any potential biases about your gender.

This is where learning how to give yourself validation and discern between true social acceptance and the projections of others becomes important. It is about learning how to choose yourself vs. waiting for others to choose you!

Waiting for social acceptance of your gender identity before you can accept yourself is an illusion. It is an illusion based on individual perceptions of what gender is. When people "accept" you, they are accepting their own projection of what gender means to them.

When you show up for yourself and put yourself first, as authentic as you are able to be, without waiting for others to accept you, you are standing rooted in your inner knowing.

You are sending energetic signals to others that you know who you are; that you don't need approval or permission slips from others to own your authentic self.

This isn't about being alone! Or pushing people away. On the contrary; this part of discernment in choosing yourself is about signaling to others that you, first and foremost, know how to depend on yourself. Know how to give acceptance and validation to yourself without the need to cling to others.

This energy signaling, in turn, attracts like-minded people. Like-minded people are independent at their core, wanting to be around equally independent people. This eliminates the need for co-dependency or any neediness for attention. Independent people don't have time for that.

Neither do you! Learn how to show up authentically and watch as the right people come into your life.

Chapter 7

Confidence Trumps "Passing," Health Trumps All

Being seen as the binary gender of male or female in society is commonly known as "passing." It's important to note that not everyone cares or strives to pass. It is equally important to acknowledge that passing matters to others and for some, it is essential for their safety.

However, when passing becomes an ideal you must reach, it can quickly turn into chasing the binary gender presentation down the rabbit hole of the ideal.

And while it is OK to have a particular look you are trying to achieve, one needs to draw a fine line between realistic aspirations vs. unrealistic ones.

Your line needs to be grounded in the awareness of your reality and your circumstances, such as:

- how many years your body has been exposed to estrogen or testosterone
- your genetics

- changes you are able to experience on hormones
- your overall health
- your access to resources, such as health insurance

Chasing that which is unachievable given your situation or context will end up eating away your self-confidence and self-worth and will destroy your mental health.

Now imagine this: What if the goal of gender transition was not to pass but to be a healthier version of you?

Think about it! What if you shifted your goal from passing to health while striving for realistic possible results? Imagine how much confidence you'll cultivate and how much happier and healthier you will become.

Chances are you started gender transition because dysphoria was eating away at your health, bit by bit. You didn't begin this path because you were striving to pass. Passing became part of the transition goal once you started, but initially, your health mattered the most.

Trust me, I know just how much passing matters to so many. And if passing is a serious safety concern, it's important always to put your safety first. But if you are overly focused on passing at the expense of your health, you risk a different side of your safety.

The path toward your authentic gender identity has much to do with balance; part of that balance is managing realistic expectations.

Chapter 8

Regrets are Just Perspectives

ne of the biggest regrets I hear is:

"I wish I had transitioned sooner."

This is especially common for older folks who step into gender transition later in life. For those whose goal is not to transition, a common regret is:

"I wish I started to explore my gender sooner."

The funny thing about regrets is that you know you can't change the past, yet you can't help but continue to dwell on it.

Regrets have always fascinated me because they are tied to a perception of a missed opportunity. For you, it is tied to the idea of missing out on doing things sooner. But what if you didn't miss out on an opportunity at all?

As a psychologist, it is my job to understand how your mind works, especially the various mechanisms it will employ to protect yourself from potential danger.

Now consider the possibility that you waited this long to explore your gender or start gender transition because that's exactly what you needed to do to protect yourself.

This is especially true for older adults. Think back to the environment in which you grew up. Do you genuinely believe it was possible to explore your gender or begin gender transition at that time? Was it safe? Did you have as many resources accessible to you as you do today?

Many of you had to work to create the financial buffer you have today to afford the gender-affirming surgeries you want or have health insurance to cover the cost.

Others needed to be more resilient to go through all the challenges gender transition brings.

Regrets are simply perspectives—a way to understand and see your life differently. Regrets are not here to make you feel guilty or sad about the past, they simply can't. Only you can make yourself feel this way.

Regrets are here to help you realize that the way the past unfolded carries its own significance. To help you trust that your starting point happened at the exact right time, it needed to happen to help you become who you are today.

Chapter 9

Rejection is Redirection

The fear of rejection, especially for trans and nonbinary folks who are older, is a big one. At the beginning of the gender transition, the fear of being rejected by your family and friends often dominates your thinking.

This fear of abandonment and not having a love of those close to you is common for so many! Sometimes, people even decide to forgo transition to avert confronting this fear head-on.

For some of you, as you get close to completing or have completed the gender transition, the fear of rejection is tied to dating and relationships.

> *"What if nobody will love and want me as a trans person?"*
> *"What if I end up all alone?"*

Such questions often prevent you from taking a risk and facing the dating arena.

One of the reasons you fear what you perceive as rejection is that you see rejection as a personal attack on who you are. That's why you often feel as if the rejection is personal. In truth, it is nothing more than discernment from the person you face.

Think about it. When you go on a date and decide the person you are sitting across from is not your match because your values don't align, are you rejecting them? Is it personal? Or are you simply exercising discernment in acknowledging they are not a right fit for you?

All of us have preferences. Boxes to check off. Lists we carry within our heads. They are there as a way to help us make decisions, even if we are sometimes quick to judge a book by its cover.

Understanding and seeing rejection as nothing more than discernment opens up a door to gratitude. Gratitude that your date exercised discernment and honored your and their time by doing so. The time that you can now invest in others who are a better match for you.

Once you understand that rejection is nothing more than discernment, you can see it as a gift of redirection. As an opportunity to course-correct in which direction you want to go.

Seeing rejection as redirection can be applied to any situation involving others. Let me give you an example. Say you have come out to your family, and some of your family members expressed discernment that they do not support you or want to be a part of your life.

A painful reality that happens to many trans and nonbinary folks. If you continue to see this incident as a rejection, it will drain your energy and leave you feeling depressed. You'll feel powerless in your life and will sink into a victim mindset:

> *"That's because I am trans."*
> *"I am defective."*
> *"If only I wasn't like this."*
> *"No one will ever love me."*

As you continue to think these thoughts, you cultivate self-loathing and begin seeing yourself as worthless.

That breeds resentment toward your own gender identity as you continue to blame your authentic self for what you perceive as rejection. Before you know it, you feel anger and frustration toward your gender and your transition goals.

But what if instead of seeing your family's discernment as a personal rejection, you saw it as a redirection? Take back your power and self-agency and correct the course you are on by acknowledging:

> *"These people will not be present for this part of my life. This is my opportunity to course-correct my path and seek those who will support me."*

Notice how I said they won't be present for "this" part of your life! That's because it's important to realize that just because your family expressed they can't be there for you now, does not mean they won't be there for you later.

Viewing this from a lens of redirection empowers you to shift direction. It puts you in the driving seat of your life and your choices. It opens up a pathway for others who want to be there for you.

Redirection is powerful! It's an opportunity! Picture your gender exploration and gender transition as a board game of life. As you come out and face people who say they cannot be there, do you throw your arms up and give up? Or do you see a blocked path on your course and redirect your movement in a different direction, opening up new opportunities for yourself?

Whenever you feel "rejected," sub the word with "discernment." Appreciate that those who exercise their discernment toward you give you a gift to invest your energy elsewhere.

Chapter 10

Cut the Umbilical Cord of Shame and Guilt

Many of you have experienced gender dysphoria starting in early childhood. Those who don't recall earlier childhood memories often experience repression, a psychological response to something unpleasant.

For example, if you are confronted with something about yourself that you find unbearably shameful, and for many, it is often tied to their gender identity, the option is to banish it from awareness, to pretend that it doesn't exist. For this reason, many adults become aware of gender dysphoria later in age while carrying traces of early childhood memories buried deep in their psyche.

As a child, one of the natural things that you try to do is to express yourself. You try to get more in touch with yourself because you are not yet influenced by the restrictions of how one should look, behave, and act, later imposed on you by society and the world.

As a child, you try to show up in the world as you see yourself to be on the inside, as well as how you see yourself in relationship to your gender.

You put on clothes that you feel define how you see yourself on the inside. You walk, talk, and behave the way you see yourself. You play by enacting gender roles you feel resonate with you. You are eager to have your parents, siblings, friends, and teachers witness your authentic self.

If you grew up in an environment where expressing your gender was not allowed, was seen as inappropriate, or perhaps you grew up with parents who held a belief of strict gender norms, it would take one look of distaste, disapproval, or disgust from a parent to spin you into repression.

One look! Even if your parents at that moment had no intention of hurting you, the projection of their inner beliefs cut like a sharp knife.

> *"What are you doing? That's disgusting!"*
> *"Why are you wearing girls'/boys' clothes? That's*
>   *not OK."*
> *"Stop behaving this way, it's inappropriate."*
> *"Why can't you act like a normal child?"*

Any of these phrases will be enough to start making you feel shame and guilt toward a part of yourself that you resonate with and a part of yourself that defines who you are.

Shame and guilt are two powerful sides of the same coin that are often used interchangeably but mean different things.

- Guilt: a feeling of responsibility or remorse for some part of your behavior, whether it is real or imagined. For example:

  "I feel guilty because I did something bad."

- Shame: a painful feeling arising from your consciousness of something dishonorable or improper. For example:

  "I feel shame because I am bad."

As a child not fully understanding the difference between shame and guilt, it is easy to internalize such things and start seeing them as a part of oneself. For this reason, a linkage is created between your gender identity and shame and guilt as you continue to perceive this part of yourself as something bad that needs to remain hidden.

To not lose the love and affection of your parents, you begin pretending to be someone you are not so that you can please them because you were too young to understand otherwise. Without being fully aware of what you were doing, you told yourself:

  "If I just try to please my parents, if I just try to be a good kid, if I just try to stay out of trouble, they will love me and never leave me."

So the cycle of pleasing others to be loved and not feel abandoned begins at an early age. You begin hiding and keeping part of your authentic self concealed to attempt to please people around you, fearing they will abandon you once they know your truth.

The longer the cycle continues, the longer you keep yourself hidden as internal shame and guilt continue to accumulate and you start believing these things about yourself.

This cycle is what I call an umbilical cord! You are attached to people around you as you keep on pleasing them in hopes of love and acceptance.

As you grow up, you continue to carry your umbilical cord attached to the people you are in a relationship with. Fearing abandonment, you take on a tremendous amount of responsibility for others in an attempt to please them.

To top it off, as you become an adult, you realize that the big part of the world and society you live in does not want to accept your true self. Thus, the cycle intensifies, and you begin experiencing low self-worth and low self-esteem as a person.

When gender dysphoria intensifies, taking hold of your health and life, the pressure to choose between yourself and your umbilical cord attachment becomes hard to bear. This is why it is so difficult for so many to own who you are.

Learning to cut the umbilical cord of shame and guilt is difficult, but it can be done!

It all starts with acknowledging that the origin of the umbilical cord that started with parents and caregivers is nothing more than a projection of how others feel about gender norms.

Once you acknowledge that, you can begin disowning ideas and perceptions of others and start owning and internalizing your own ideas of who you are.

Note that you can't cut the umbilical cord until you can start valuing, loving, and caring about yourself. This may sound easy, but it is very difficult to do when you have spent years and years loathing yourself.

To begin cultivating a self-loving practice, acknowledge your needs and wants. Take time for yourself and write down what it is that you really want to bring into your life. Your wants and needs can be as big as starting to deal with gender dysphoria and as small as buying yourself flowers.

Once you have your list, you can start bringing these things into your life. This is what I call learning how to be "healthy selfish" by finally doing the things you want vs. what others want you to do.

Learning how to love yourself is a daily practice filled with gratitude and space to honor your being. It's not easy, and you will experience a lot of resistance because it will feel foreign and unfamiliar to you to suddenly do things that you desire.

But it will get easier and when it does, it will be your time to finally cut the umbilical cord of internal shame and guilt.

To be free, you must be self-determined, which is to say that you must be able to control your own destiny in your own interests.

— Stanford Encyclopedia of Philosophy

ON YOUR TERMS

Chapter 1

Redefine What Gender Transition Means to You

One of the biggest challenges are the words gender transition themself. Transition implies the process or period of changing from one state or condition to another, suggesting a set destination point and a linear process from segments A to B.

I prefer gender evolution because you are evolving into a more authentic version of yourself. Evolution also suggests an ongoing process as you evolve into different versions of a changing self.

The idea of core gender identity that never wavers nor shifts in expression and presentation doesn't exist. Sure, for many, there is a stable core gender identity. However, even the core is mutable throughout one's life and expresses itself in many ways that may depart far and wide from the core identity.

For example, a trans woman with a female core identity, masculine gender role, and feminine expression. Or a nonbinary person with a fluid gender identity, feminine gender role, and masculine expression.

Your sense of self expands as you go through life and accumulate experiences. Changing and shifting internally and externally. All life experiences create a new way of being and a new way of experiencing yourself about your gender.

This is why it is important to redefine what gender transition means to you, and to establish your personal path of your evolution toward your truest self.

There is no one way to go through gender transition. There is only your way, and it is you who needs to define it.

Anyone who claims you must begin with a social transition and move on to hormones or have all the surgeries is lying. There is no linear progression in gender transition, nor are there milestones you must meet, except your own.

Chapter 2

Surgeries and Hormones are Not Mandatory

M any people still believe that identifying as transgender or nonbinary means you must go through a gender transition. That the transition process must entail hormone therapy and surgeries.

Wrong!

This misconception stems from the view that trans and nonbinary people struggle with crippling body dysphoria and, as a result hate every body part. There is also a myth that one is not "trans enough" if one decides not to have genital surgery. Such ideas continue to perpetuate the idea that there is only one way of being in this world as a trans or nonbinary person.

In reality, there is a multitude of options depending on your personal goals and your circumstances:

- deciding to abstain from hormone therapy due to potential health risks

- deciding to take hormones only for a short period of time to achieve the desired changes one was looking for
- unable to take hormones due to health concerns, lack of access to resources, or financial hardship
- deciding to abstain from surgery because hormone therapy alone aided in achieving congruency
- deciding to have some surgeries to feel more aligned but not genital surgery due to potential surgical complications
- deciding to not have genital surgery because one doesn't feel genital dysphoria and enjoys genital intimacy
- unable to pursue surgery(s) due to health concerns, lack of access to resources, or financial hardship

Apart from this, there are many other options people choose from. Remember, hormone therapy and gender-affirming surgeries are there to aid in modifying your secondary sex characteristics to help you feel aligned with your gender identity.

Hormones and surgery do not define your gender identity—you do. These are simply tools to help you feel more aligned, if you need to, with your gender. But your gender identity, essence, and spirit are internal and only felt by you internally.

What's mandatory, in my view, is for you to live your life as close to who you are as possible. To show up in the world in the spirit of who you truly are, with or without the aid of hormone therapy or gender-affirming surgeries.

Chapter 3

Stop Giving Others Your Pen

When making your own decisions in your life, especially about your gender identity, you write your own story. When you write your own story, you own it, including full copyright to the script.

Doesn't that sound powerful? I bet it does!

Life unfolds as one big story of your life. From the moment you were old enough to make your own choices, you began writing your script.

Sure, some things happen in your life that are beyond your control. But you do have control over how you internalize and understand the experiences that happen to you—most importantly, the choices you make.

I see so many people walking around with their life manuscripts, eagerly passing them around to others; family members, friends, co-workers, partners, and even people on social media one has never met.

People offering ownership of the pen that writes the manuscript so they can write their version of you in your story.

Ask yourself, am I permitting everyone around me to write in my storybook? If you answered yes, don't worry; there is ample time to take full ownership of your story and rewrite where your main protagonist is headed.

And if you are still hesitant to fully own your story, imagine this: It's the end of your life and you are invited to a screening of your story. Sitting in the theater, popcorn in hand, you eagerly await the start of your life movie, only to find out it is no longer yours!

Suddenly you see parts where your mom edited your script, inserting her ideas of your gender identity. As the movie unrolls, it shifts from person to person as you watch your siblings, co-workers, and even your partner, edit your thoughts because of how *they* see you in your story!

Which version would you rather watch?

A mosaic of many voices of how you ought to be, all coming from projections and opinions of others? Or would you rather witness a distinct story that is true to who you are?

Even if your story is filled with challenges, obstacles, regrets, and unfulfilled dreams, it is still yours! It belongs to you and no one else!

Stop giving others ownership over your pen. Stop allowing others to define and write your story. Stop giving up your copyright to who you are. Own it. Claim it. Live it.

Chapter 4

Collect Your Own Stars

Feeling self-worth and a sense of inner value is essential for your healthy life. Without it, you fall victim to co-dependency and unhealthy entanglements with others.

The need for self-worth is ingrained into us. We are all social creatures living within social interactions with others. We all need to feel valuable.

Especially at the start of the gender exploration or gender transition, many of you may experience a high desire to feel worthy of others. As the desire persists, you begin searching for it in others and suddenly find yourself needing more of it.

That's because your golden stars (remember those stickers you got in school for doing well) representing your self-worth are given to you by others instead of you giving them to yourself.

When a sense of self-worth of who you are constantly comes from the outside, it leaves you empty. A co-dependency is created. You find yourself needing that person all the time to make you feel valued.

Now imagine what would happen if the golden stars came from within. If you had an unlimited reserve of stickers inside of you and could give yourself one, two, or three, anytime you felt a need for it?

Owning a set of your golden stars is called having a healthy reserve of self-worth. It is a way you value yourself. It is knowing and feeling that you are worthy. And while it is OK to have others gift you golden stars, there is nothing compared to an internal drawer full of your own.

That's why it is important to collect your own stars, to start a daily practice of cultivating your self-worth.

How do you do that? Notice your inner dialogue. What does it sound like? Is it negative, hateful, or self-deprecating? The roots often start with how you talk to yourself and hey, I have my moments too.

The key is to keep overall inner chatter positive. No, I am not talking about just positive thoughts, although that helps. I am talking about beginning to value yourself as a human being worthy of living and experiencing happiness.

I know that years spent living with shame and guilt of who you are, are hard to eradicate. But it is possible.

You can also begin acknowledging things you feel confident or good about. It could be your professional life. Your role as a partner. Your ability to parent. Or your overall integrity as a person.

Realize what you already value about yourself and notice how you have a multitude of things to feel worthy about.

Start small and watch as your stars accumulate. Believe in yourself and your potential. If there are things you objectively think can improve, focus on how you can improve them, and before you know it, you'll be giving those gold stars to yourself.

Chapter 5

Learn How to Die Empty

When I tell my clients to learn how to die empty, I am often met with confused looks on their faces.

"Die empty?"

Assuming I am implying to die without meeting their dreams, goals, and desires to be who they truly are. Then I pose a question I read in Todd Henry's *Die Empty* book:

 What do you think is the most valuable land in the world?

What answers come to your mind? The Middle East? Or the riches of Africa? Perhaps it is the rising capital of California in the US?

Well, as it turns out, the most valuable land in the world is the graveyard!

Yup, the cemetery.

The cemetery is where all the unwritten novels, never-started businesses, never-created ideas, never-expressed gender identities, and authentic expressions of self are buried!

The most common phrase we all utter is:

"I'll get around to that tomorrow."

Daily. Hourly. Often several times a day. Until one day, the day you were planning to get to, the day you were thinking of starting to own who you are, runs out.

One thing we can all agree on is that death is inevitable. We also have no knowledge of when it is coming to claim us. And yet so many of us live each day as if we have an unlimited amount of life.

Dying empty is a gift you can give yourself. It is a gift to yourself and to life itself. Dying empty means you lived! You brought riches from within into the world instead of burying them deep into the ground.

To learn how to die empty, start a vision board. Vision boards are an incredibly powerful visual tool as they help externalize your dreams and desires through images. You can make various vision boards representing each dream you have.

- vision board of how you see your gender identity, presentation, and expression
- vision board of your personal aesthetic and clothing style
- vision board of things you value about yourself and things you want to bring into your life
- vision board of how you envision your life in your authentic gender, where you work, travel, and play

Interestingly, when I ask my clients to create a vision board of how they see their gender identity being represented, about 80% of the time, that's exactly whom they evolve into.

Now that's what I call a visual manifestation of the self!

Go ahead, learn how to die empty! Set your dreams free and watch them fly!

Chapter 6

Stop Apologizing

Your gender is not an apology. Let me repeat that: your gender is not an apology. Neither is your existence. Your desire to better your health and well-being. Your wish to be happy.

And yet so many continue to apologize for being who they are.

Coming out, apologizing:

> *"I am sorry, but I am transgender."*

Asserting your pronouns, again, apologizing:

> *"Sorry, but you got my pronouns wrong."*

Experiencing being misgendered, yup, apologizing again:

> *"Sorry, but I am nonbinary."*

Sorry, sorry, sorry, sorry.

When you apologize for who you are, you indirectly negate ownership of your gender identity. Without realizing it, you communicate to the other person that you feel sorry for your existence.

Saying sorry conveys that you did something wrong. That's what the apologies are for. To make amends. To let another person know that whatever you did, was not right. That you are guilty. A bad person.

When it comes to your gender identity, saying sorry communicates to others that something is wrong here, which is not true. There is absolutely nothing wrong with your gender identity. So please, stop apologizing and start owning who you truly are.

Self-acceptance is an essential step. It is more crucial than any other steps you may take. That's because self-acceptance resides at the core of your being.

Like a nucleus, it takes residence at the depth of your inner self, from which all your relationships and interactions with the world occur.

But what is self-acceptance? Most importantly, how does one get to the point of integrating this concept into your life?

Simply put, self-acceptance is your satisfaction or happiness with yourself. Self-acceptance involves understanding who you are. This understanding comes from awareness of your strengths and weaknesses.

Only after looking at your strengths and weaknesses can you step back and accept all aspects of yourself—those parts you see as bad, good, desirable, and undesirable.

Self-acceptance doesn't mean you want things to change. Nor does it mean letting go of the pain and hurt you may feel.

Instead, self-acceptance is stepping into the now and seeing things as they are. It is accepting things about yourself without judgment, shame, guilt, or any other negative feelings you tend to attach to yourself.

I know that for many trans and nonbinary folks, self-acceptance is often a challenging step. It might feel difficult to achieve, but it is possible.

The first step toward self-acceptance is to claim what is yours. Even if you strongly feel you didn't ask to have gender issues or to be born with gender dysphoria, it still doesn't change the fact that it belongs to you. Your gender is always yours to claim.

You don't need to apologize to anyone for who you are, whether you see what you are going through as a blessing or a curse.

You are not a burden. You are not a pariah. You are not a sick person. You are not delusional or mentally ill.

You are a human being who is either struggling with gender dysphoria or is on their way to exploring their relationship to gender.

You subconsciously dehumanize yourself by not claiming this part of who you are. As a result, you subconsciously message others that it's OK to dehumanize you:

> *"Because you see, I am not human, and I am not worth it."*

Stop disowning a big part of who you are! Claim it. Claim all of you! Without judgment, shame, guilt, or hate. Just as is.

Once you claim a part of yourself you have been disowning, you are ready to own it. Ownership means you have the power and control to choose what to do. Owning parts of yourself lets you decide what's best for you and your well-being.

Ashleigh Brilliant said:

 I may not be perfect, but parts of me are excellent.

Talk about a great example of what ownership looks like.

Healing begins when you no longer cast away parts of yourself you find undesirable, and start owning who you are.

Finally, you are ready to begin unapologetically living after claiming and owning who you are.

This final step in self-acceptance is about letting your actions speak louder than your words. In this step, you begin living by following your truth. Your vision. Your representation of who you are. Authentically showing up in the world and claiming your space.

These steps toward self-acceptance don't just happen overnight. Neither is it a linear process.

Self-acceptance looks different for everyone. Self-acceptance is an ongoing practice. It takes time. Dedication. Patience. It takes compassion and self-love to master self-acceptance of who you are, but I promise it's worth it.

Chapter 7

Know When to Draw a Line

Boundaries are an essential part of your well-being. They are necessary if you want to preserve your sanity and mental health.

But did you know there is more than one type of boundary? And that boundaries can range from being rigid to permeable.

Enter your boundary tool kit! I like to consider this tool kit as an internal council of advisors. Each represents a boundary type to protect your inner queen or king from harm. Yes, very medieval of me, I know.

Whether you realize it or not, you already have some boundaries in place. What you may need to know is just how variable each boundary is.

- Emotional: there to protect your own emotional well-being.
- Physical: to protect your physical space.
- Sexual: protecting your needs and safety.

- Material: there to protect your material belongings and surroundings.
- Time: protecting the use or misuse of your time.
- Intellectual: there to protect your thought processes.
- Workplace: protecting your ability to focus on work without interference or drama.
- Gender: protecting your gender identity.

Did any of these surprise you as being boundaries?

Boundaries can be anything that matters to you at any given moment for which you would like to draw a line. You may even have a set of boundaries not listed here for which you have elected an inner council member to protect you.

Boundaries are not only variable based on your individual needs, they also vary based on the setting. Think about boundaries as an ability to regulate the flow of information, resources, people, and energies into your space. This means your boundaries can be:

- Firm: clearly define what is OK and not OK for you. Firm boundaries, while being firm, are often open to flexibility.
- Flexible or permeable: boundaries open to cross but under certain circumstances.
- Rigid: nonpermeable, nonflexible boundary or think wall, drawn up to protect you, period.

Boundaries can also vary from time to time. You may draw a boundary line today and remove it tomorrow.

As you are going through a gender transition, boundaries become even more critical. That's because you are more likely to dismiss yourself and your well-being and focus too much on how others feel around you. Fearing hurting others and being abandoned, you neglect yourself. In an attempt to protect others, you end up hurting yourself.

While it is important for all of us to be mindful of others, it is even more important for you first to consider what's a priority concerning your health. It won't serve your loved ones in the long run if you suffer and struggle to protect them.

So rally up, get your council members together, and decide which area of your life needs support, protection, and extra space to allow you to focus on yourself. Put boundaries in those places. Modify when a need arises. And trust that your loved ones can handle their own feelings.

Chapter 8

Ultimatums are Rigid Corners of Others

Receiving an ultimatum is common if you are in any relationship, be it romantic, a friendship, or a professional relationship.

Ultimatums are often seen as a final demand of terms, the rejection of which results in a breakdown of a relationship.

Let's look at ultimatums in detail. For starters, there is no win-win when it comes to ultimatums. No room for negotiation or compromise. It is a rigid boundary of one person, often intending to maintain the status quo.

Ultimatums are not open to flexibility. Nor are they open to discussion of possibilities and changes to the current structure of the relationship.

I say they are rigid corners of others because that's exactly what they are—inflexible, sharp edges with only one outcome in mind.

To the receiving person, ultimatums often feel selfish or not fair and that's because they are just that. The person demanding an ultimatum is acting in their self-interest, clinging as hard as they can to maintain the current parameters of the relationship.

Keep in mind that not all ultimatums remain rigid, especially those within a long-term marriage or a relationship. For example, it is very common for a long-term partner to issue an ultimatum as soon as you come out.

With time, the rigidity of the ultimatum becomes more flexible and open to new dynamics in the relationship. In fact, there is a pattern: the longer your relationship is, the more likely an ultimatum will follow.

As humans, we tend to be risk averse; a tendency to avoid the risk associated with a perceived loss of something we value. For this reason, your partner looks at the scope of the relationship as an investment and becomes very territorial when a possibility of loss arises.

If you find yourself in a long-term commitment and you come out, chances are your partner will throw an ultimatum in the form of:

> *"If you decide to go through gender transition, I leave."*

Sadly, for many other couples, the ultimatum maintains its rigidity. There is no room for openness, leaving a person to decide between health and marriage.

If confronted with an ultimatum, consider just how rigid and impermeable the boundary is for that individual. If the boundary is fixed with no possibility for change, it's a sign that you need to start thinking about your well-being.

Chapter 9

Don't Annihilate Your Inner Ruler

I f you are familiar with my work, you'll know that I am a big proponent of integrating elements of your past with your present. That's because there is a psychological reason for it.

A life spent in the gender you were assigned at birth, even if it did not align with you, accumulated experiences. These experiences shaped your character, defined your personality, and determined your temperament.

As you go through gender transition, deciding to negate the past part of your life as if it did not happen to you is akin to splitting your headspace in half.

Visualize your headspace as a kingdom. The person sitting on the throne, your king or a queen, is your Ego. The Ego is a part of you that presides over the kingdom of your mind. It is the part that makes most decisions about your life.

To illustrate, let's say you were assigned male at birth, but your inner core identity is female. For a part of your life under the king (for simplicity's sake, I am sticking to the male/king, female/queen dichotomy) regime, the landscape of your head-space is shaped by experiences you have accumulated as you lived your life in this gender.

These experiences stem from how people interacted with you based on the gender you were assigned. The decisions you had to make. The careers you decided to go into. The relationships you committed yourself to.

Every interaction, every relationship, and every encounter constitute your subjective reality. Everything you have ever experienced is added to the intricate design of the landscape of your kingdom.

Now, as a king, looking over your surroundings, you can see some inauthentic parts of the design, masqueraded as male-ness, you never connected with.

Of course, there are parts of your surroundings that will remain true to you no matter what your gender identity is.

The way you love. How you give. Your ability to nourish. These and many other characteristics will remain the same.

Thus, your kingdom combines an authentic you and a pretend you into one big landscape.

As you become aware of your feminine gender identity, it becomes her time to take over the throne. A new queen to be crowned! A new ruler to rule over the kingdom.

Sadly, I often see how quick people are to bring down prior rulership. To annihilate their inner ruler, to overthrow the king. To attempt to destroy the complexity and depth of the psychic landscape they created.

Instead of annihilating your king (or queen, or however you see your royalty), I suggest an integration—a merger of the two.

To begin with, it is important to acknowledge that your former ruler kept you alive amidst dysphoria. For many of you, your inner ruler kept you employed and provided necessities such as food and housing. For those who are older and lived when being trans was unsafe, the ruler kept you alive.

And as much as you may not like the gender the ruler identified with at the time, it is important to acknowledge that it sustained your life so that one day, you could live an authentic one.

The integration begins with gratitude—a big thank you.

Next comes the time to claim your throne. This is the time when you allow your authentic self to rule over the kingdom.

At this point, you may feel eager to siege, imprison, or even kill, your previous ruler. To which I say NO!

Instead, take the opportunity to practice integration. A practice where you allow your demoted king to stand behind your new queen; silently, and open to the queen's aid may she need knowledge of the intricate design of the kingdom as she reshapes her new territory.

Speaking of which, this is the time to redesign and redecorate your landscape. Notice how some parts of the previous regime will remain, as there will always be genderless pieces of who you are. Or perhaps you decide to keep things from your past that align with your present.

Learn how not to annihilate your inner ruler. Learn how not to destroy everything you have built up to this point.

Integrate by taking over the throne in your truth and authenticity. Command over your future from the seat of authority, empowerment, and ownership. Redesign your inner landscape and in doing so, you will begin to redesign your life as it unfolds in front of you.

Chapter 10

Learn How to Live in the Now

I t is important to learn how to live in the *now*! Not tomorrow, not yesterday, *now*. After all, now is all that you have.

Yesterday is already gone, and tomorrow is not yet here. The only changes you can make, the only shifts you can bring to your life, are present now.

Someone once said that thinking about the past is living in depression. Thinking about the future is living in anxiety. Thinking about the present is living mindfully.

Living in the *now* allows you to control your time, current day, and current situation, especially when it comes to gender identity and the overwhelming anxiety you feel about the future. You know, all those things you ruminate about:

> *"Will I get desired changed on the hormones?"*
> *"How soon?"*
> *"What will others think?"*

"Will I get misgendered?"
"Will I be attractive?"
"Will others like my name?"
"What will they say when I come out?"

Gender transition will also stir up depressive feelings if you think about the past.

"I should have started sooner!"
"Why didn't I call the clinic last month?"
"I should have come out last week."
"I should have made a therapy appointment weeks ago."

All of these thoughts are designed to weigh you down. Imagine each thought from the past and the future weighing 5 lb. The more thoughts you have about things you should have done or fears of how they will unfold, the more weight you add to your carrying load.

The reality is that you already have a mountain in front of you, whether you are exploring your gender, thinking about starting a gender transition, or wherever you are in your gender journey.

Because the truth is, living authentically is climbing a mountain. That mountain is you! Your life!

Adding additional weight is masochistic. And I feel you don't want to do that to yourself.

Learn how to live in the *now*. Learn how to release the past because it is no longer here. Learn how to let go of the future because it has not yet come. All you have is the *now*.

Be yourself; everyone else is already taken.

— Oscar Wilde

Acknowledgments

Like any big life moment, gender transition, the birth of a child, or losing a parent, writing a book is one of them and it's a process involving many people.

Mom, thank you for always having my back and always being there. Thank you for holding space for me to entertain my dreams.

Helen and Julia, thank you for always being my biggest cheerleaders.

David, thank you for your love, support, and attention as I think through my ideas.

Thank you to every person I worked with intimately, allowing me to hear your stories.

Thank you to every viewer of the video content I produce and everyone who has interacted with me via comments. Your stories shaped the tapestry of this book.

Tara Solomon, thank you for all the copyedits, proofreading, and suggestions that improved this book.

Marko Polic, thank you for making my vision a reality by creating the book cover.

And thank you to the muses who danced around me till I finished. May you never leave me.

Bibliography

Ahmed, Sarah. (2006) *Queer Phenomenology.* Duke University Press.

American Psychiatric Association. (2022). *Diagnostic and Statistical Manual of Mental Disorders.* (5th ed., text rev.). https://doi.org/10.1176/appi.books. 9780890425787

Barres, Ben. (2018) *The Autobiography of a Transgender Scientist.* Cambridge, MA: MIT Press.

Beckwith, Michael. (2013) *Life Visioning: A Transformative Process for Achieving Your Unique Gifts and Highest Potential.* External Dance Music.

Brené, Brown. (2012) *Daring Greatly: How the Courage to Be Vulnerable Transforms the Way We Live, Love, Parent, and Lead.* Avery Publishing.

Butler, Judith. (1990) *Gender Trouble: Feminism and the Subversion of Identity.* New York: Routledge.

Coelho, Paulo. (2006) *The Alchemist.* HarperOne.

Eckhart, Tolle.. (2008) *A New Earth: Awakening to Your Life's Purpose.* Penguin: Reprint Edition.

Ettner, Randi., Monastery, Stan., and Coleman, Eli. (2016) *Principles of Transgender Medicine and Surgery.* Second Edition. New York, NY: Routledge

Fausto-Sterling, Anne. (2012) *Sex/Gender. Biology in a Social World.* New York, NY: Routledge.

Fausto-Sterling, Anne. (1987) *Myths of Gender: Biological theories about Women and Men.* New York, NY: Basic Books.

Fine, Cordelia. (2010) *Delusions of Gender. How Our Minds, Society, and Neurosexism Create Difference.* New York, NY: W. W. Norton & Company, Inc.

Gherovici, Patricia. (2010) *Please Select Your Gender: From the Invention of Hysteria to the Democratizing of Transgenderism.* New York, NY: Routledge.

Gherovici, Patricia. (2017) *Transgender Psychoanalysis: A Lacanian Perspective on Sexual Difference.* New York, NY: Routledge.

Gree, Jamison. (2004) *Becoming a Visible Man.* Vanderbilt University Press.

Gozlan, Oren. (2018) *Current Critical Debates in the Field of Transsexual Studies.* New York, NY: Routledge.

Gozlan, Oreng. (2015) *Transsexuality and the Art of Transitioning.* New York, NY: Routledge.

Halberstam, Jack. (2018) *Trans. A Quick and Quirky Account of Gender Variability.* Oakland, CA: University of California Press.

Harris, Adrienne. (2009) *Gender as Soft Assembly.* New York, NY: Routledge.

Hawkins, Sterling. (2022) *Hunting Discomfort: How to Get Breakthrough Results in Life and Business No Matter What.* Wonderwell.

Hendricsk, Gay. (2010) *The Big Leap: Conquer Your Hidden Fear and Take Life to the Next Level.* New York, NY: Harper Collins.

Henry, Todd. (2013) *Die Empty: Unleash Your Best Work Every Day.* Portfolio.

Hillman, James. (1996). *The Soul's Code: In Search of Character and Calling.* New York, NY: Warner Books.

Hillman, James. (1999). *The Force of Character and the Lasting Life.* Random House.

Jacobs, Denise. (2017) *Banish Your Inner Critic: Silence the Voice of Self-Doubt to Unleash Your Creativity and Do Your Best Work.* Mango Publishing Group.

Jeffers, Susan. (2007) *Feal the Fear and Do it Anyway.* New York, NY: Random House.

Jung, Carl. (1997) *Jung on Active Imagination.* Princeton University Press.

Kabat-Zinn, Jon. (2005) *Wherever You Go, There You Are: Mindfulness Meditation in Everyday Life.* 10th ED. Hachette Books.

Kishimi, Ichiro. (2018) *The Courage to be Disliked: The Japanese Phenomenon That Shows You How to Change Your Life and Achieve Real Happiness.* Atria Books.

MacKinnon K., Kia H., Salway T., et al. Health Care Experiences of Patients Discontinuing or Reversing Prior Gender-Affirming Treatments. *JAMA Netw Open.* 2022;5(7):e2224717. doi:10.1001/jamanetworkopen.2022.24717

Lev, Star Arlene. (2004) *Transgender Emergence: Therapeutic Guidelines for Working with Gender-Variant People and Their Families.* Binghamton, NY: The Haworth Clinical Practice Press.

Lorber, Judith. (2022) *The New Gender Paradox.* Cambridge, UK: Polity Press.

Paoletti, Jo. (2012) *Pink and Blue: Telling the Boys from the Girls in America.* Indiana: Indiana University Press.

Pressfield, Steven. (2002) *The War of Art: Break Through the Blocks and Win Your Inner Creative Battles.* New York, NY: Black Irish Entertainment LLC.

Richardson, Sarah. (2013) *Sex Itself. The Search for Male & Female in the Human Genome.* Chicago: The University of Chicago Press.

Rubin, Rick. (2023) *The Creative Act: A Way of Being.* Penguin Press.

Russ. (2019) *It's All in Your Head.* Harper Design.

Serano, Julia. (2016) *Whipping Girl: A Transsexual Woman on Sexism and the Scapegoating of Femininity.* Berkley, CA: Seal Press.

Sinek, Simon. (2009) *Start with Why.* London, UK: Penguin Books.

Stockton, Kathryn Bond. (2021) *Gender(s).* Cambridge, MA: MIT Press.

Vanderburgh, Reid. (2007) *Transition and Beyond: Observations on Gender Identity.* Portland, OR: Q Press.

Winfrey, Oprah. (2019) *The Path Made Clear: Discovering Your Life's Direction and Purpose.* New York, NY: Flatiron Books.

Woodman, Marion. (2001) *Bone: Dying into Life.* Penguin Books; Reprint Edition.

About the Author

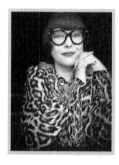

Dr. Natalia P Zhikhareva, known as Dr. Z, is a clinical psychologist specializing in working with transgender and nonbinary adults, a writer, and a motivational speaker.

Dr. Z's commitment and dedication to helping people become the person they most want to be led to the creation of DR Z PHD YouTube Channel. Her direct and analytical approach brought her an ever-increasing following, drawn to her ability to understand gender dysphoria in its full depth.

Dr. Z regularly writes blog posts featuring the latest information on gender-affirming medical care and is often featured discussing gender issues on podcasts and interviews.

Her private practice, DR Z PHD, is set up to support transgender and nonbinary adults who are struggling with gender dysphoria, unsure of how to take first steps, and those who are ready to transition, need direction or wondering if it's worth it for them.

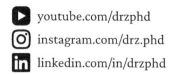

youtube.com/drzphd

instagram.com/drz.phd

linkedin.com/in/drzphd

Printed in Great Britain
by Amazon

20415988R00079